Birgit van Damsen

INSECT PROTECTION
for Horses

Tips and tricks

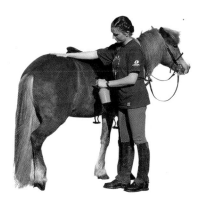

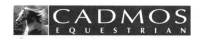

CADMOS
EQUESTRIAN

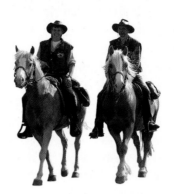

Contents

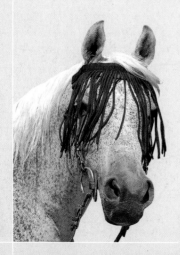

Imprint

Copyright © 2004 by Cadmos Equestrian
Copyright of original edition © 2003 by
Cadmos Verlag
Translated by Desiree Gerber
Project management by Editmaster Co Ltd
Design and composition: Ravenstein, Verden
Photographs: Birgit van Damsen
Printed by: Grindel Druck
All rights reserved. Copying or storage in
electronic media is permitted only with the prior
written agreement of the publisher
Printed in Germany.

ISBN 3-86127-943-6

A little entomology

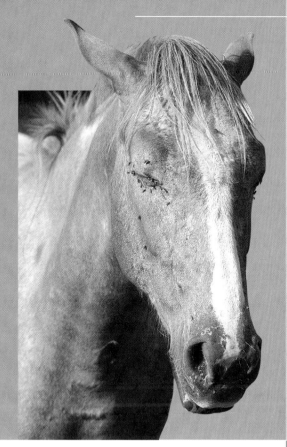

The months between April and October can be extremely difficult for horses, due mainly to the enormous amounts of insects buzzing around. The various types of insects not only make life trying but also spread bacteria, viruses, worms and other parasites. They also trigger allergies, infect wounds and cause inflammation of the skin and mucous membranes. Horses that are out in the paddock twenty-four hours per day are especially at the mercy of these pests.

Horses try to rid themselves of these pests by twitching muscles, swishing the tail, shaking the head, stamping their feet, rolling, scratching, biting and mutual grooming; they sometimes even flee, panic-stricken. A long tail and thick mane will offer some comfort, but caring owners will proffer additional safeguards to protect their horses against flies, midges and ticks.

Unprotected horses in the paddock are at the mercy of insects

On the basis that to fight an enemy, you must first understand it, we shall discuss the different insects in terms of their appearance, how they breed, when they are around and how they affect our horses.

Rolling in the dust helps to keep insects away.

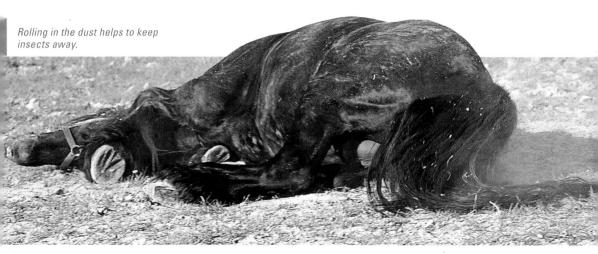

Flies

Both the small and the common housefly count as genuine flies *(Muscidae)*. They are 5–7mm long, have two wings, short feelers and a proboscis to dab with. They lay their eggs mainly in droppings, muck heaps and spilt food rests; the eggs hatch within a few days.

Houseflies are around mainly from June till October, and are especially busy in the afternoon. They use their proboscis to lick and suck at the moisture around the nostrils, eyes or any broken skin of the horse. While doing so they pass on bacteria and the larvae of worms, directly to the skin of the horse, and cause all types of wounds that do not heal.

The 5–6mm-long biting fly is related to the stable fly. The stable fly *(Stomoxys)* lives mainly in stables, where it also breeds, while the biting fly can be found mainly on pastures from June to September. Both these flies prefer horned animals, but will also burden horses that are living in close proximity to cattle. These flies have a prominent proboscis with which they administer nasty bites to their victims. They carry many pathogens, like contagious anaemia, that are then passed on to other animals.

Horse-flies *(Tabamidae)* also suck blood. These are the tough, bristly flies, with big eyes and biting probosces. Horse-flies are up to 25mm long and are indigenous to Europe.

The bites of the female horse-flies are incredibly painful and can cause sustained bleeding. This will in turn attract the normal stable flies. The emerald green horse-fly is especially active on warm, muggy days, whereas the

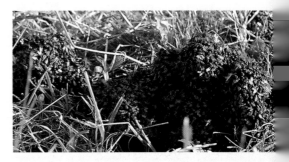

Horse manure has magical powers of attraction for flies.

Flies and worms multiply without restraint in unkempt paddocks.

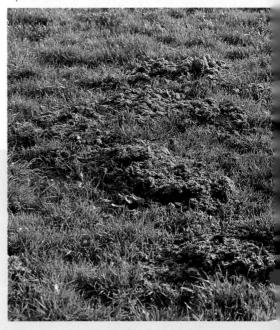

Flies are often the cause of running eyes. The resulting liquid from the eyes attract even more flies.

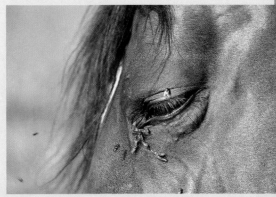

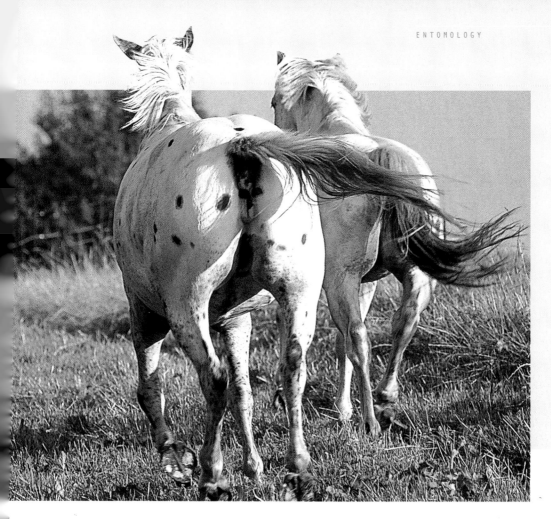

Many horses will flee in panic when horse-flies draw near to them.

grey rain horse-fly will bite even in cloudy and drizzly conditions. Horse-flies are active from late morning well into the evening. Due to their blood-sucking activities, horse-flies play a major role in spreading various diseases. One of the diseases they can spread amongst humans is infectious anaemia. In India the horse-fly spreads a highly dangerous horse fever known as Surra; in South America it spreads lameness of the loins (mal de caderas).

The 11–13mm-long horse bot *(Gastrophilus intestinalis)* lays its eggs on the legs of the horses in the months of June up to September. The screwworm fly *(Rhinoestrus purpureus)*, which is indigenous to Eastern and Southern Europe as well as North Africa, will in contrast lay its eggs in the nostrils of the animals. One will occasionally find the screwworm fly in our latitudes between August and September. They can cause mucous and throat infections as well as coughs and head shaking. Even though the depositing of the eggs causes no physical pain, most horses will react with strong resistance and flight reactions.

The hatched larvae irritate the skin and prompt the horses to lick the area. In this way the larvae arrive in the mouth and burrow into the tongue, resulting in inflammation of the mucous membranes, the tongue and the gums, and difficulty with chewing and swallowing. In the next three to four weeks the larvae will migrate to the stomach of the horse and bring about inflammation of the stomach wall, colic and diarrhoea. The mature larvae will be passed through the faeces within the next eight to ten months, develop into a pupae in the meadow and hatch in no more than four weeks. The female fly will start to lay her eggs directly after the mating process. The only sure way to interrupt this cycle is to treat the horse with a wormer in autumn in order to kill off all the larvae. Additional methods of reducing the larvae include proper paddock management (removing all manure), as well as the physical removal of the bot eggs from the horse's legs. The eggs can be recognised as small yellow-white spots that cling to the hair. One can wash them out of the hair with relative ease by applying a mixture of water and cider vinegar, or by scratching them off with a razor blade, in the direction of hair growth – never against the hair!

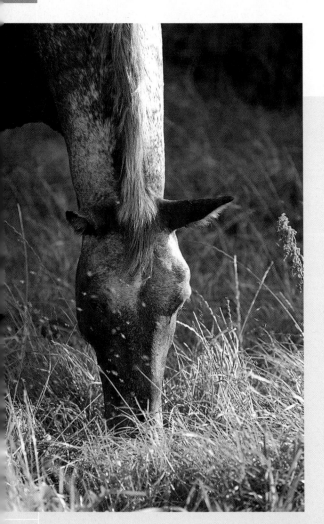

Swarms of midges buzz around horses at dusk.

Midges

Midges are the second largest group of insects that pester our horses in the summer months. The mosquito families are included in this group. It is only the female insects that bite. These reproduce in and around the water's edge in ponds and other damp areas, and are for the most part active at dawn or dusk in areas protected from wind.

Midges are generally slim, thin-legged with two wings and biting-sucking mouths. The best-known amongst the mosquito families *(Culicidae)* is the nasty common gnat *(Culex pipiens)*. The females hibernate through the winter months in cellars and houses and lay eggs on the water in springtime, where the larvae hatch within three weeks.

Swarms of these nasty midges buzz around at dusk, the females typically close to the ground. Amongst the significant biting midges is the 10mm-long banded mosquito *(Theobaldia annulata)*, found close to polluted water, the

6–9mm-long snowpool mosquito *(Aedes commu-nis)*, whose larvae live in shallow pools in wood-land, as well as the 6mm-long inland floodwater mosquito *(Aedes vexaus)* that can become a real nuisance in marshland. The midges not only cause irritating itches, but can spread various diseases. In horses they can spread infectious anaemia and Onchocercariose (ringworm).

The 3–6mm-long blackfly *(Simuliidae)* is a small, fly-like midge that lays eggs in running water and appears in large numbers in the areas of brooks and fluvial plains. Blackflies are a menace for animals in the paddock, their poisonous bites damage the heart and circula-tion and can even affect the respiratory sys-tem.

Water is the breeding ground for midges.

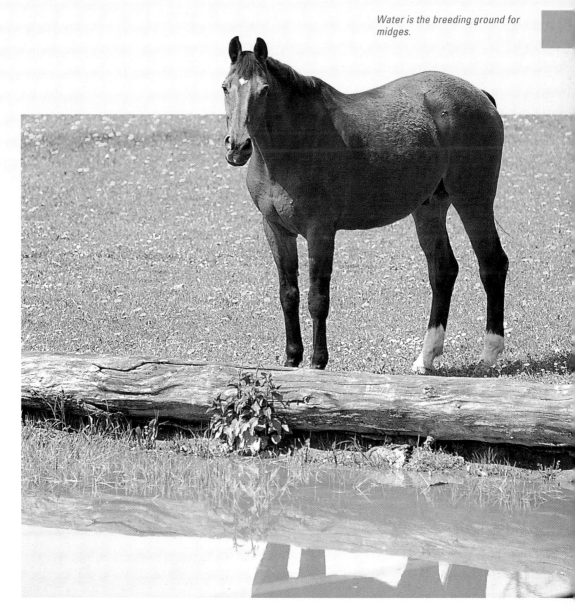

In severe cases an exceptional number of bites can lead to poisoning and even death. In the twenties and thirties of the 20th century, an especially deadly blackfly caused havoc in the Balkans, killing thousands of animals on the pasture, amongst them many horses. As a rule the bites of the blackfly in our region merely cause itchy lumps, mainly in areas where horses have little or no hair.

A further unpleasant bloodsucker is the tiny 1–3mm-long midge *(Culicoides)*. These pests prefer wind-protected damp areas, where they also lay their eggs. Midges are active from May to October, more so in the warm and humid spring and summer months. Their main activities occur at dawn and dusk, two to three hours after sunrise and two to three hours before sunset. Their bites contain an anticoagulant (prevents blood clotting) that itches like mad and triggers an allergic reaction that leads to the feared summer eczema, also known as sweet itch.

These small midges prefer to crawl into the manes and dock of the tail, but will also go for the croup, as well as under the belly towards the udder or sheath, the withers, ears and eyes.

If the horse has an allergic reaction, the bites will create swelling under the skin. This itchiness will induce the horse to rub the areas, thus causing eczema-like conditions on the skin, with loss of hair, pimples and crusty areas, sometimes leading to bigger wounds.

Sweet itch can occur in all breeds of horses and is a separate illness that should not be confused with other types of skin disease with similar symptoms, for example worms or fungal infection, mineral or vitamin deficiencies, mite infestation, fleas and even lice. A definite diagnosis can be given with the help of an allergy blood test in a specialised laboratory. Unfortunately it is not possible to de-sensitise the horse. Various therapies will treat the symptoms, but none will treat the reason for the allergy. Swiss and Swedish scientists have been working on vaccinations against insects.

Until a vaccination is found, the only way to avoid or reduce the symptoms is to take preventive measures in the fields of feeding, stabling, insecticides and protective clothing, as well as making use of the many medicinal possibilities.

The bites of midges are incredibly itchy

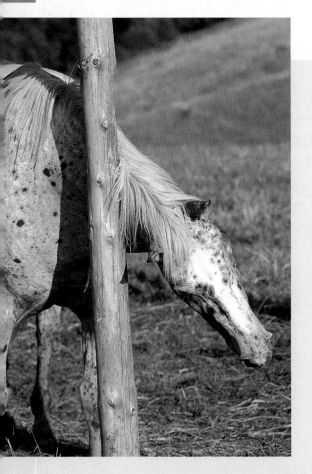

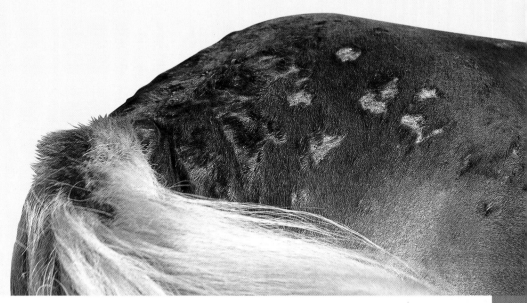

*Excessive scratching can
cause eczema of the skin*

Ticks

Ticks, which have eight legs, do not belong to the insect family, but to the mite-like parasites. From the worldwide 890 species of ticks, the most significant ticks in Europe are the forest ticks and the nasty sheep tick *(Ixodes ricinus)*. The sheep tick favours light foliage and mixed forest where they lurk in the undergrowth, on small shrubs and high grasses, waiting to pounce on their unsuspecting victims. The tick season lasts from May until October, but the blood-sucking parasites are especially vicious from mid-May to mid-June, and again from mid-August to mid-September. The tick bite itself is not painful but will merely cause a light itch. The tick is, however, equipped with a mouth-part that has anchoring organs, covered with backward curving hooks that they use to attach themselves to the skin. The preferred areas where the ticks bite are on the inside of the hind legs, the fold of the elbow and the dock of the tail. This does not mean that the chest, neck, coronet, nostrils and eye region will escape without harm.

Even as a larva the tick carries bacteria in its salivary gland. The asexual nymph obtains these bacteria from the blood of rodents, for

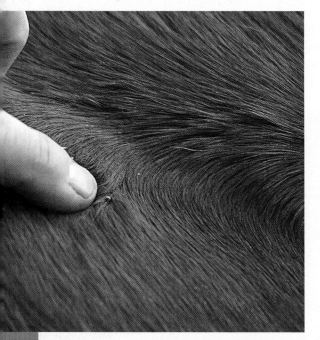

Initially the ticks are minute, therefore the horse must be thoroughly inspected.

Removal of a tick with the use of tick removal forceps.

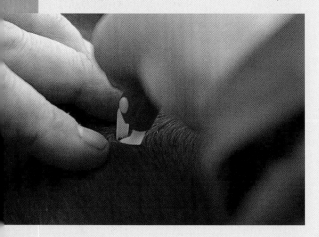

lymph nodes. Epidemic babesia is also caused by tick bites. A type of equine meningitis has also occurred in the USA.

The biggest danger, however, lies in Lyme disease, which attacks the nervous system, for this disease is incredibly difficult to diagnose and treat. To date there is no protective vaccination available for man or horse. Tick repellent cannot offer a sure safeguard against ticks, and the best prevention is the rapid removal of the tick and disinfection of the bite. The tick should never be simply pulled from an animal, for the head, the carrier of the disease, will be torn off and stay put in the skin. Crushing or squeezing oil or an adhesive on the tick is also of no avail, for, in its death throws, the dying blood-sucker can secrete an enormous amount of poison into the bloodstream of the horse. Ticks should only be removed with special tick removal forceps, available from your vet or pharmacy. Using these forceps, the tick is seized as far to the front as possible, and gently pulled from the skin. It is not necessary to twist the forceps to achieve this.

Horses in paddocks that border on woodland or paddocks where many shrubs grow are in greater danger from ticks. All horses should be checked for ticks after riding in a forest with undergrowth. Ticks also attack humans and it is therefore advised that the rider inspects him- or herself after such a ride, especially if they were lightly dressed.

example mice, and will inject it into the blood of the host as a sexually mature female.

These bacteria transfer dangerous diseases. In humans this can cause meningitis and Lyme disease. In horses it can cause localised sepsis and allergic reactions with swelling of the

Prevention and protection in the way we keep and feed horses

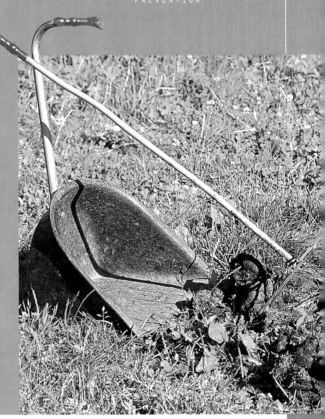

Unfortunately it is close to impossible for the normal horse owner to stamp out all insects from the stable and paddock. Insect levels can, however, be dramatically reduced by taking proper hygienic and protective measures.

The location and even the time when the horses are allowed on the paddock will furthermore be crucial to the total annoyance caused by the insects. Not least of all, a balanced feed with special additives can add to the protection of the horse, from the inside.

Droppings must regularly be removed from the paddock.

Stable and paddock hygiene

When the stables, exercise areas and paddocks are kept immaculate, the breeding cir-

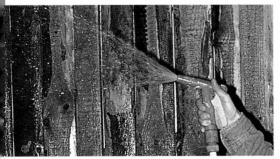

Washing and disinfecting the walls and floors of the stable on a weekly basis will reduce the insect population.

cumstances will be minimal for the insects. Stable hygiene should consist of daily mucking out and regular disinfection of the stable floor.

Shavings are more suitable as bedding in the summer months owing to the fact that it is easier to see and remove the soiled shavings. With straw, on the contrary, urine and droppings always remain and will therefore attract flies. The horse should, however, always have good quality hay available as feed.

A big contribution to daily stable hygiene is the removal of feed rests and cleaning of the water containers. Feed and water troughs should be washed with lemon juice or vinegar on a regular basis, for this will also help to keep the insects under control.

Removal of droppings from the paddock twice a week (daily is better) will prevent excessive reproduction of flies and worms.

The manure heap should, if at all possible, be located as far away as possible from the stables and paddocks, and preferably be covered with a plastic sheet.

In view of the fact that midges prefer moist areas to reproduce, it is important to remove puddles, sludge or other damp patches, either by drainage or by covering them with sand. There are also special products available in the trade that can be mixed and spread on all the possible breeding spots of insects, for example marshes, manure heaps and so forth. If this is done in the winter months it will dramatically reduce the insect population in summer.

Protective devices in the stable and paddock

A well-tried method of repelling flies is to whitewash the walls of the stables. Sprayed lavender oil, or a lemon covered with cloves, will also assist in keeping insects at arm's length. Another method is to employ fly papers in the stable. The rolled strips of fly paper are coated with a special glue that attracts flies, which then adhere to the stickiness.

Fly traps suspended roughly 15 metres outside the stable in direct sunlight are an additional, extremely effective preventive strategy. The bait, which is free from poison and not dangerous to beneficial insects, humans or domestic animals, will attract flies into a pouch. A trap will ensure that the flies cannot escape again.

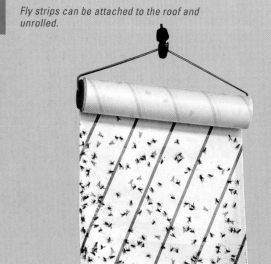

Fly strips can be attached to the roof and unrolled.

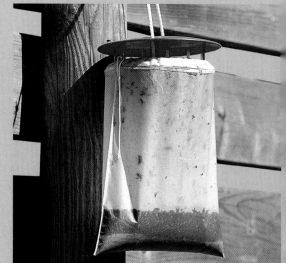

Solar vaporisation will distribute the fly catcher's odour in the atmosphere and draw the insects.

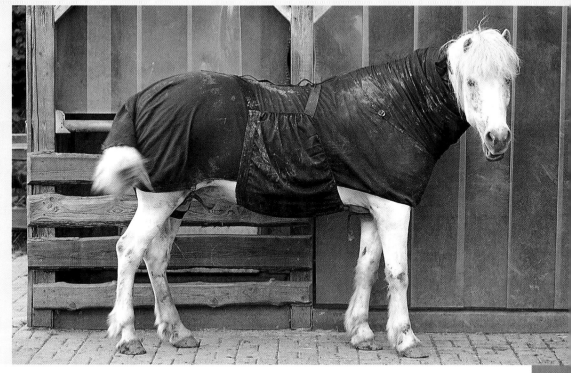

Horses that are prone to allergic reactions are reliant on an insect-free zone being created

This bait is active for a period of four weeks and the insect population can be reduced considerably in this time. The plastic top can be used more than once and the pouch is degradable.

The methods outlined above are no help against mosquitoes. Ultra violet light attracts all the mosquito types, and an electric insect destroyer can consequently be successfully employed against them. These electrical appliances can be placed in the stable, provided they are well out of reach of horses. The blue UV light attracts the mosquitoes and they are then eliminated via protected electrical bars.

Attaching netting to the windows or doors of the stable can be helpful against bigger nuisances like the flies, biting mosquitoes and horse-flies. Smaller insects like gnats and midges, however, can crawl through this netting. Strips of transparent plastic have proven successful as curtains in front of windows, doors and entrances to open stables and huts in paddocks. These overlapping plastic strips are extremely effective in repelling insects. The strips should be let down one at a time in order to allow the horses to become accustomed to them.

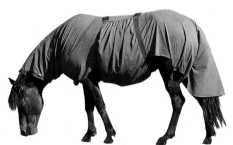

Tip:

■ ■ ■ ■

Spiders are first-class helpers against insects. They catch a variety of insects in their freshly spun webs. Old, however, as they are no longer effective.

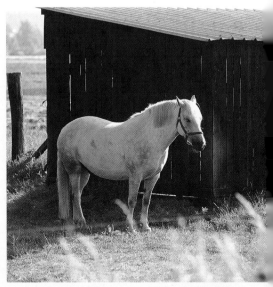

The ichneumon wasp or fly is nature's best biological weapon against flies in the stable. It eradicates the larvae of the flies, is not dangerous to humans or horses, as it does not sting them, and spends most of its time at the manure heap. These beneficial insects can be bought in containers and introduced to the manure heap. Advertisements for these insects can be found in the classified sections of specialist magazines.

Horses must be protected against insects in the paddock. While horses will retire to the protective shelters at dusk, they prefer to doze in the shade of trees in the heat of the day. This time of day is when flies are active. If the paddock has no trees or other shelter, mobile shelters are always an option and a good solution, as no planning permission is required to move them into the paddock.

Various shrubs can be planted to assist in the protection against insects in the paddock. The robust and fast-growing elder bush is known for its strong perfume, which permanently drives away insects.

Horses doze in shady, breezy spots in the heat of the day.

Brushes, broom heads and wooden posts hold no risk of injury when horses rub against them.

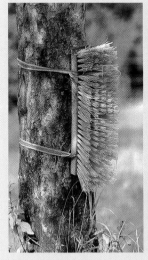
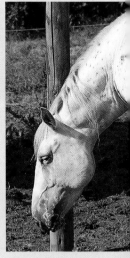

Sharp or splintering objects and low-hanging branches should be removed from the stable and fenced in on the paddock, to prevent horses with sweet itch from scratching and wounding themselves.

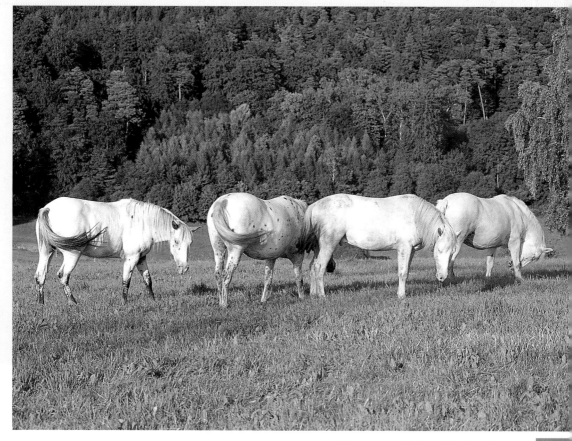

*Horses on paddocks at the edge of a
forest are more vulnerable to insects*

The horses should nevertheless be provided with an alternative scratching device. Smooth, solid wooden posts and properly fixed brushes or broom heads provide ideal solutions for this predicament.

Location of the paddock and the best time to turn out

The location of the paddock can be crucial with regard to insect plagues. Paddocks at the edge of a forest, close to flowing or standing water and damp valleys will always be prone to higher levels of insect nuisance.

Paddocks such as these ideally should be used in the spring (but watch out for ticks near forests!) or autumn only. Due to the excessive occurrence of mosquitoes near water, paddocks near water are completely taboo for horses with sweet itch. These horses should, where possible, only be kept in more airy paddocks, for example on elevated ground.

The time when the horses are turned out also plays a significant role in protecting them against insects. The best turnout time (for a horse with sweet itch) is from nine am until four pm in the spring and late summer.

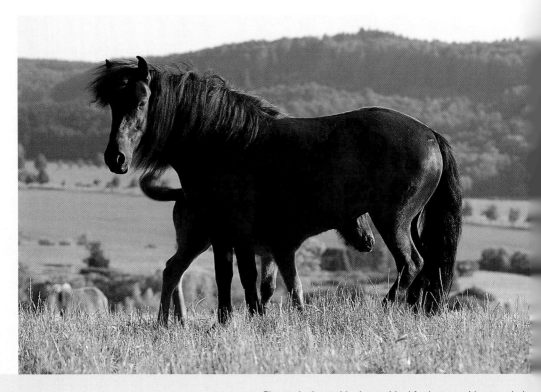

Elevated, airy paddocks are ideal for horses with sweet itch.

Horses often prefer to stay in the stable when insects are a major nuisance.

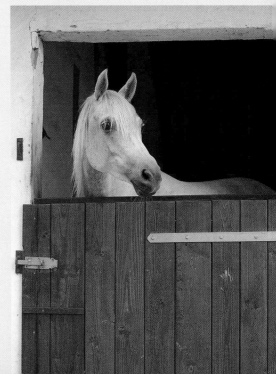

During the midday heat of high summer, it is sometimes best for horses with sweet itch or an insect or pollen allergy to be turned out at night, when it is completely dark.

Horses that are predisposed to sunburn will also prefer to graze at night. In principle, all horses should have shelter in the paddock and the allergy susceptible ones should have extra and appropriate protection against insects. If such protection cannot be provided, the horses should be stabled during the affected hours.

Prevention through feeding

Insect protection from the inside means that horses are fed balanced meals, with sufficient minerals, trace elements and vitamins but not excessive protein or energy. This is especially important for the allergic horse, for the intestines play an integral part in the immune system, with the allergens being dismantled and excreted from the intestinal tract. When the intestinal flora are out of balance, the resulting disturbance in the metabolism can encourage skin problems such as sweet itch. For this reason a feed with low energy and protein levels (sparse grass on the paddock, little hard food, abundant fibre) with individually adjusted vitamin and mineral requirements, is the optimal solution for horses predisposed to eczema. Supplements to strengthen the immune system of the allergic horse are out of place in this situation.

The allergic horse should be fed merely to regulate its immune system and to stimulate good metabolism. This includes for example linseed, which promotes digestion and protects the mucous membranes of the intestinal tract. Silica has a positive effect on dry and itchy skin, improves the elasticity of the skin and in particular promotes skin metabolism when combined with zinc and seaweed. Various plant oils can be fed to support the natural functions of the skin, for example caraway or horse chestnut oil as well as herbs such as nettle leaves and burdock roots.

Pressed or chopped garlic (three to six cloves daily) is an excellent supplement to mix into the horse's feed, and can be fed to all horses, not just those which have problems with allergies.

Garlic can also be bought from feed distributors in granule and pellet form. It is particularly effective when combined with vitamin B.

Tip:

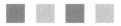

It is recommended that you consult with a feeding expert before adding any feed supplements, and if need be have the blood tested for any shortages.
Most supplements can be changed or interrupted between feeds if required.

The smell of garlic will repel insects.

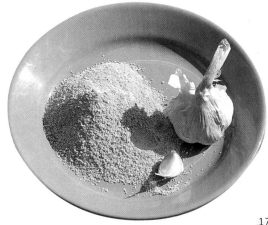

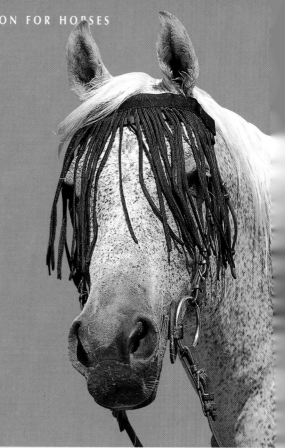

Protective equipment

There are many varieties of protective gear that will safeguard a horse's head and body from insects when grazing, working or dozing. These are freely available in tack shops and in the classified section of magazines. In principle one should pay attention to individual fit, quality of the material used, craftsmanship and horse-friendly buckles and clips of the equipment when buying. Good quality is more expensive as a rule, but is more sturdy and enduring and probably equipped with tried and tested features.

Protective headgear

Brow band fly fringes have demonstrated sufficient shielding for simple protection of the horse's eyes against flies. They are often manufactured from leather, nylon or cotton and have various methods to attach them to the head collar or bridle.

Brow band fly fringes are best suited for riding and driving. In the paddock it is often the case that less experienced horses get into trouble with these fly fringes. They might catch a branch on the head collar that is a necessity with such a fly fringe, or get tangled when scratching their faces with the hind legs. It is therefore recommended that security halters

with Velcro fastenings, or fly fringes with built-in headpieces, are used in the paddock. These are held in position around the poll and throat with thin straps that will tear in emergencies. The strap under the throat can also be replaced by an elastic band.

Horses that have sensitive ears can wear cotton fabric hoods that cover the ears with or without fringes. This is an ideal solution when riding, fitted under the bridle onto the poll piece.

The best protection against flies is a complete mask that covers both the ears and the eyes, manufactured of fine nylon netting. These masks are available in different sizes and should be of good quality.

Simple netting that is only attached to the horse's head with thin fabric strips is not recommended, for it will not close tightly enough to stop insects from crawling in under the cloth. Protective masks with padded edges and Velcro fastenings, or elasticated features and even drawstrings with security clips, are much more reliable in the field of protection against insects. Full-faced black netting masks will offer sanctuary against the rays of the sun for sensitive eyes and head-shakers, as well as protection against insects, all without compromising eyesight.

More recently the market also offers a new cover for the nostrils of head-shakers or those horses prone to sunburn. Made from dark material, they will safeguard the horse's nose from sun and insects, without affecting its breathing. This nose cover is available in two sizes and can be attached to the halter or bridle with Velcro strips.

Special hoods for horses with sweet itch can be made from breathable fabric to protect the whole head from small midges.

1 Nylon brow band fly fringe attached to the bridle.
2 Leather fly fringe attached to the head collar.
3 Cotton fly fringe with home-made elastic band.
4 Ear hood under a driving bridle.
5 Blackfly mesh with secure fastenings.
6 Complete hood for horses prone to eczema.
7 Simple netting mask with straps.

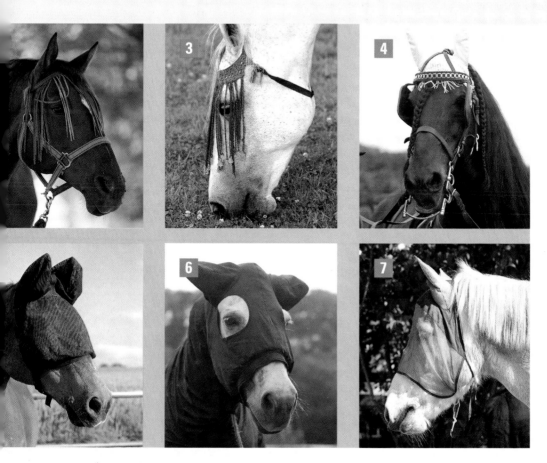

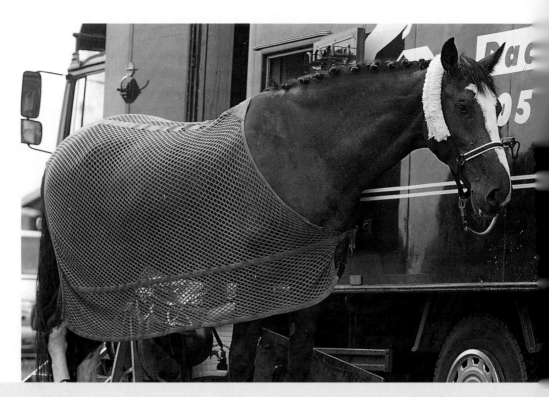

Cotton sweat rug.

Fine mesh polyester rug

Rugs

Rugs for protection against flies are available in various fabrics, with a variety of sizes of mesh. Cotton sweat rugs with large mesh, also put into service as protection for the kidneys, shield riding and driving horses from insects when they are sweaty, whilst at the same time allowing the air to dry the skin. Such rugs are suitable for and often used in competitive situations.

Similar rugs, manufactured from fine polyester netting with a single buckle or clasp at the front, are also available. When the horse wears one in the paddock, an extra elastic belly girth and temporary crupper must be fitted. A

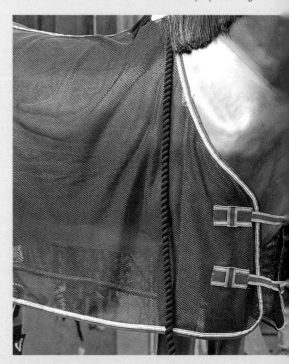

rug without these extras can become entangled in the horse's legs when it rolls, which can lead to injury of the horse or tearing of the rug.

There are also netting rugs made especially to wear in the paddock, with integrated belly straps, tail and leg straps, that offer proper protection and will stay on the horse. These rugs are manufactured of lightweight breathable PVC or polyester material and are available with or without additional neck cover and UV-protection. All-over covers are available for horses that suffer from eczema, with neck, belly and tail flaps. These rugs are normally manufactured from breathable, waterproof material that dries quickly, is robust and can be cleaned easily.

Elastic features around the neck and stomach flaps will be more reliable in insulating the horse from insects. It is however important that these rugs fit well, and do not impair the horse's movement or influence social contact. Rugs that fully protect the horse are now freely available in the trade. Some manufacturers even offer made-to-measure and repair services.

All-over rugs are a sure protection against insects.

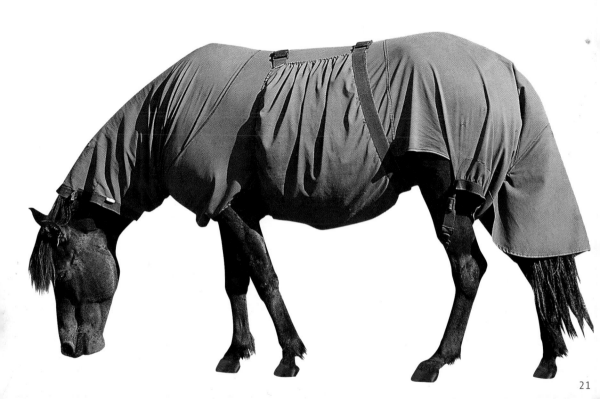

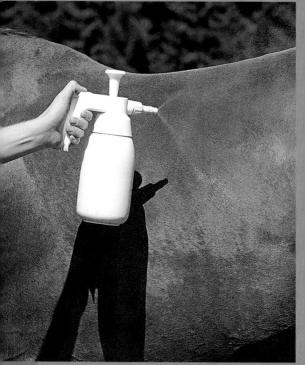

Many repellents can be sprayed on the skin of the horse

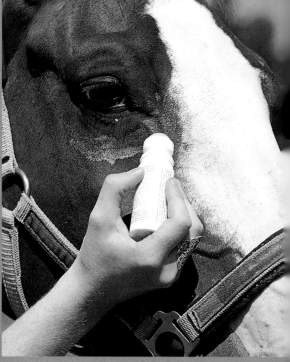

A roll-on is a good way to apply insect repellent around the eyes.

Insect repellents and cleaning products

Insecticides, which kill insects, as well as chemical and natural repellents, the so-called deterrents, are all classified as insect repellents. Furthermore, there are diverse cleaning products that have added anti-itching, calming and anti-inflammatory effects. After all, damaged skin and mucous membranes must be treated and protected against insects.

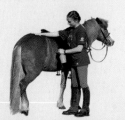

Insecticides and repellents

Insecticides contain the active ingredient Permethrin, a poison derived from pyrethrum found in the chrysanthemum, that is damaging to the nervous system of insects, but is not dangerous for vertebrates. Despite that, some side-effects are possible when this ingredient comes into contact with wounds or mucous membranes. This poison only has a lasting effect when it is permanently in contact with the horse's skin. Insecticides are available from the vet in shampoo, powder, lotion and collar form.

Repellents are more widely available on the market. Synthetically manufactured repellents contain substances like diethyltoluamid or parallethrin.

These drugs should not be allowed to come into contact with the eyes or the mucous membranes for this can result in localised skin irritation.

In addition to that, there is a multitude of biological repellents available that are non-poisonous and are as a rule not harmful on skin. Most of these are available as a mixture of essential oils of citronella, mint, eucalyptus, aniseed, cedar wood, clove or lavender oil.

Some repellents also contain skin-caring oils and ingredients such as aloe vera, avocado, walnut and sesame seed oils.

Other natural remedies are Australian tea tree oil and Indian neem oil. These oils have a disinfecting quality and they promote healing as well. Some companies add resinous ingredients to their products that exude an odour. There are also products on the market that unite with the smell of the horse.

An alternative to essential oils and additives are all the repellents that are on the market. These repellents have added natural substances like aromatics, plant extracts, for example lemon grass and geranium and even foul-smelling animal oils. The preparations with the malodorous oils are mainly suited for the outside world of the paddock, due to the impossible smell. Take care, as these preparations may leave yellow stains on grey horses.

Repellents are either available as a ready to use spray or as concentrated lotions that have to be diluted before use. They must be sprayed or applied to a clean, groomed horse on a regular basis.

A spray is fundamentally a better idea, as this is more effective.

Tip:

A thick lotion can be mixed with some water to make it into a spray.

Pressure pump atomisers are the best to use when spraying repellents, as they are easy to manage. Although they are more expensive, the containers do last relatively long. Because the spray is so fine, it means that the lotion is conserved, making it economical as well. The spray action of the pump will not hiss like other spray cans, making it ideal for extra-flighty horses. With ample patience and copious amounts of praise, however, one can just about get any horse accustomed to a spray.

The period of effectiveness given by the manufacturers of the different repellents will vary between eight hours and two days.

Most products have to be applied more than once a day. Many of these repellents will only be effective against ticks for two hours. Sweating will also shorten the effectiveness of the product. Horses that are sensitive to the rays of the sun will not be protected sufficiently by all the products. The best protection for sun-sensitive horses is a sun protective gel for humans with a protection factor of at least 25, which can then be applied to the specific problem areas such the ears and nostrils.

There are very few products that can be applied on open wounds, soft genital tissue and the face. The manufacturers have however developed a roll-on to apply on the face, and a gel for the udder and sheath is also available.

A rich skin cream that is freely available commercially can also be used on the udder and sheath. The ears can be protected against small midges by applying a zinc ointment. These soft areas, ears and around the eyes should be cleansed with chamomile tea on a regular basis. Take care that no tea runs into the eyes or ears!

Tip:

Home made repellents:
For the paddock: Mix equal amounts of water and fruit vinegar with a shot of "Frenchman oil", available from pharmacies.

For hacking: Mix grapefruit seed extract, available from the pharmacy, according to the instructions given on the package.

For both hacking and the paddock: Mix equal amounts of water, fruit vinegar and eucalyptus bath oil with some clove or lavender oil (approximately 15 ml oil per litre mix). Essential oils must be diluted to prevent any allergic reactions and skin irritations.

Protective products

It is especially the small midges such as the gnats and the blackflies that have it in for the belly, the dock of the tail and the mane. In order to keep these insects away, as well as preventing itchiness and rubbing of the mane and tail, manufacturers have many grooming oils and emulsions on the market that will quench the itch and soothe the skin.

Apart from the essential oils, these preparations include skin stabilising and regenerating oils derived from marigold, thistle, hemp, wheat germ or avocado.

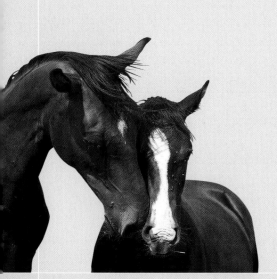

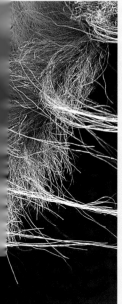

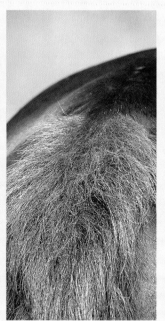

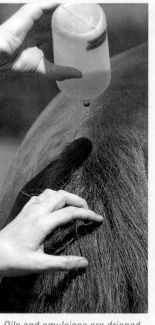

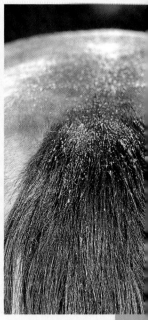

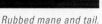
Rubbed mane and tail.

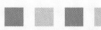
Oils and emulsions are dripped on the mane and tail and massaged in.

Sand particles can easily stick to the oily lotions..

Some remedies also contain additional anti-inflammatory substances, for example neem- and tea tree oil, and even mineral substances from the Dead Sea in order to stimulate the metabolism of the skin.

One thing all these preparations have in common is that they should be applied in good time, that is before the beginning of the insect season, and then, once the season commences, on a regular, if not daily basis, on all the appropriate areas on the body that are vulnerable.

Dust and sand particles will normally stick to oily substances on the skin once the horse has rolled, and this makes it important to wash the skin with green tea or a special horse shampoo and reapply the oils after the skin has dried.

Tip:

■ ■ ■ ■

Home made preventive caring emulsion:
Mix 500 ml baby oil with 50 drops of citronella oil, 20 drops of eucalyptus oil, 20 drops of cedar wood oil, 20 drops of clove oil, 10 ml tea tree oil and 50 ml of black caraway seed oil and rub into the mane and tail on a daily basis.

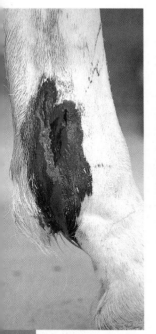

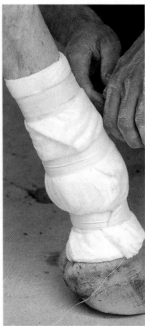

Blood magically draws flies; it is therefore better to bandage wounds such as these.

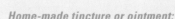

Home-made tincture or ointment:
Mix 100 ml jojoba oil when used on the mane and tail or 100 grammes of Vaseline when used on the body, with 20 drops of tea tree oil and 5 to 10 ml of chamilosan, and apply daily.

Treatment and protection of injured skin and mucous membranes

Big and bleeding wounds such as cuts and tears must be treated by a vet and shielded from insects by applying a protective bandage over the wound.

In comparison to that, superficial grazes and scratches can be safeguarded from infection by insects after thorough disinfection and then applying powder sprays or special pastes on the wounds.

Small grazes or simple eczema can be treated with lotions or even liquids containing zinc or tea tree oil. These substances have a fly repellent action as well.

In the case of an extensive graze wound or even sunburn, a paste of green clay or therapeutic mud can carefully be spread over the whole surface area of the wound. These pastes are pain-relieving as well as cooling, reduce itchiness and cover the skin, preventing the rays of the sun as well as the insects from penetrating to sensitive areas.

Open eczema can be treated with topical ointments and creams. In cases of severe and chronic sweet itch, the vet should nevertheless be consulted.

Short-term administration of cortisone and antibiotics can ease the symptoms.

Healing paste protects against germ-spreading insects; it should be checked every day.

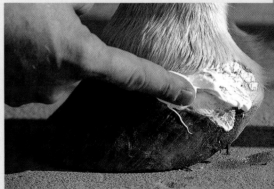

Rubbing in sweet itch oil will also help in the prevention and treatment of eczema. Homoeopathic treatment of summer eczema and head shaking is possible, but a professional practitioner must be consulted for the correct remedy and dosage,

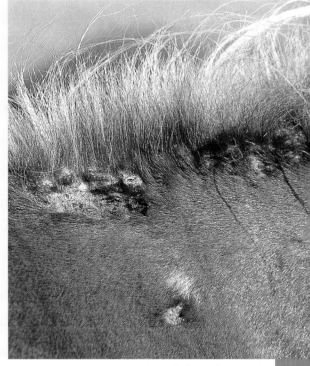

Sweet itch must be treated professionally.

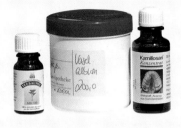

Effective remedies can be prepared from Vaseline, chamillosan and tea tree oil.

Tip:

All medication must be applied according to the instructions.
Never use more than one kind of therapy at a time, and always discuss and co-ordinate treatment with the vet.

Flies not only bring a flow of tears to the eyes of the horse, but can also cause inflammation of the eye, redness of the conjunctiva and swelling of the eyelid. This is even more a prob-lem when the horse rubs the eye or has an allergic reaction to flies. The vet must prescribe the appropriate eye drops or ointment when the horse has an infection or the eye is swollen. The eye should not be washed, but rather covered with a damp sterile pad and protected from flies with the necessary headgear.

As a rule, insect bites are not dangerous when they do not cause any allergic reaction. In theory, horses can suffer an allergic reaction to every and any insect. However, only rarely do insects cause allergic shock symptoms such as staggering, sweating, and trembling, turning it into a veterinary emergency.

Tip:

Allergy tests are available for the following insects and midges:
Storage mites, bees, fleas, house dust mites, hornets, common gnats, horse-flies, mosquitoes, stable flies, wasps, ticks, blackflies, ants, buffalo gnats.
These tests are available from specific laboratories: ask your vet for further information.

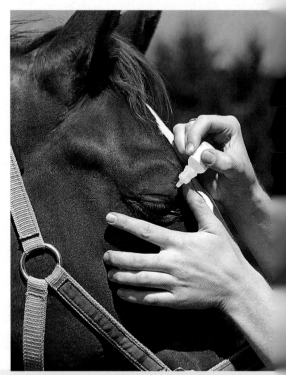

Eye drops are carefully applied in the lower eyelid.

The vet should be called when the horse has any insect bites around the eyes and in the throat area. For a horse, a swollen throat can mean choking and even suffocation. Bites that bring about such swelling are usually caused when the horse swallows a wasp or hornet while eating fallen fruit. For this reason fallen fruit should be collected, or the trees fenced in.

Localised swelling and itches can be controlled with the use of gels for human use or various old-fashioned household products that have stood the test of time. Onion juice applied on itches has a soothing and disinfecting action. Garlic also has an anti-inflammatory and soothing effect when rubbed on itchy spots, and when combined with vinegar and water, it cools the area and will reduce any swelling.

Onions, garlic and fruit vinegar aid in the relief of insect bites.

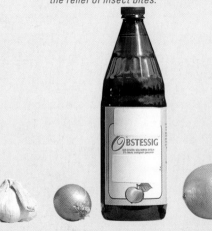

Protection when riding

Horse and rider must be well prepared for a ride in the summer months if the hack is to remain pleasurable, rather than a struggle against insects. The timing, location and speed of the ride can also have an influence on contact with insects. Grooming after the ride should be part of the overall preventive action.

What to wear

The horse can be protected from insects with a fly fringe, hood for the ears or netting over the nostrils.

Full fly rugs cannot be used when riding. The best solution against insects when riding is careful use of repellents.

The rider may also be plagued by insects when out riding, perhaps with the exception of

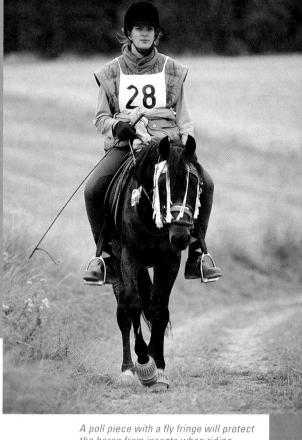

A poll piece with a fly fringe will protect the horse from insects when riding.

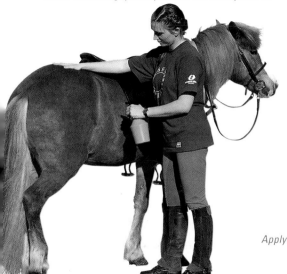

the big horse-flies, which normally only bite our four-legged friends. The rider should therefore apply insect repellent lotions on his or her own body as well. Tick bites are most unpleasant and you are well advised to wear thin, long-sleeved clothing, even in warm summer weather, and to avoid riding through thick forest or underbrush.

Apply a good layer of insect repellent on the horse before riding.

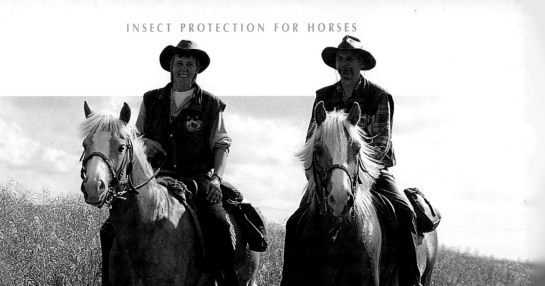

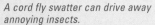

Long-sleeved shirts and hats are good protection against ticks.

A cord fly swatter can drive away annoying insects.

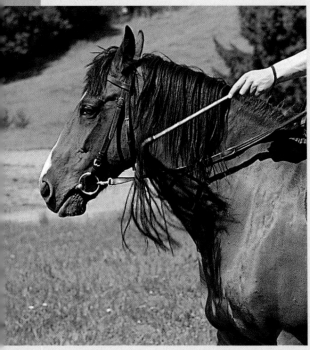

The rider can additionally carry a fly swatter. With a bit of skill, such a fly swatter can also be hand made. If needs be, a twig with some leaves or a long whip will also do the job.

Suitable time, route and pace to ride

Early morning is the best time to ride, two to three hours after sunrise being optimal. Midges and gnats retire early and at this time the horse-flies and mosquitoes, which only become active later in the afternoon, are not yet around.

The ride should be planned in advance, and areas with high insect populations, for example livestock meadows, the edges of forests, marshes, ponds and lakes, should be avoided at all costs. Higher ground is best, where the movement of air will keep insect activity to a minimum.

The smell of horse sweat has an enormous power of attraction for insects and the pace of the ride should therefore be adjusted in the warm months, for once the horses start to sweat, the repellent loses the ability to repel and the insects become a real nuisance. This means that extended cantering (and associated sweating) should be avoided when riding in the hot summer months.

Necessary grooming and hygiene

Warm and sweaty horses should be cleaned with plenty of clean water after a ride. Care should be taken that the neck, chest, saddle and girth area, as well as the region between the legs, is washed properly. Sweaty patches on the

Riding on exposed and elevated ground will keep insects to a minimum.

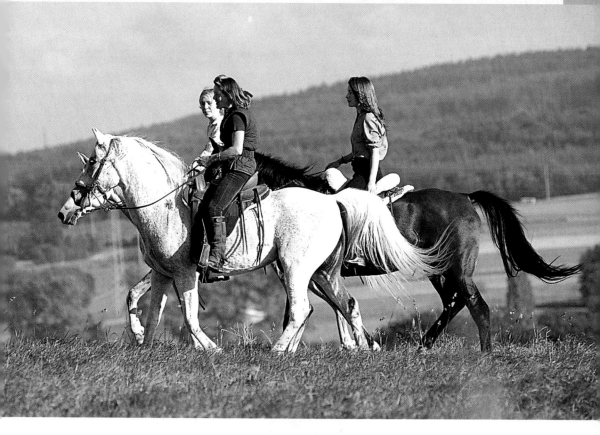

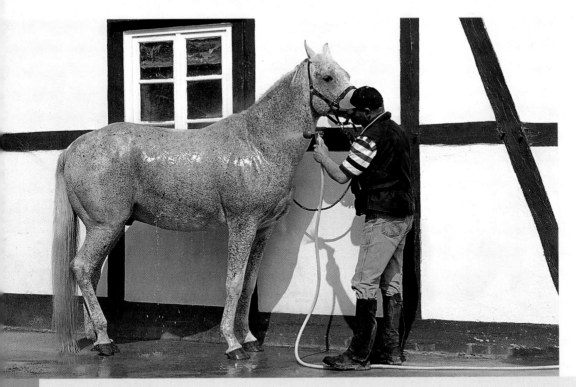

*Thorough hosing will clear
sweat from the horse.*

face can be cleaned with a moist sponge or
towel.

Once the horse has been dried, using a sweat
scraper and towel, a new layer of insect repellent must be sprayed on the horse or the regular protection, for example rug and fly fringe,
must be put on it, before it is allowed to go out
on the paddock again.

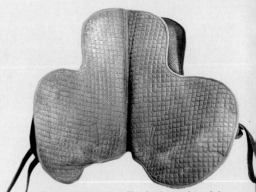

*Dirty saddle pads will ruin the action of the
repellent and must be washed on a regular
basis.*

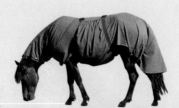